If Lost, Please Return
This Planner To:

This Week

/

/

/

/

This Week

/

/

/

/

/

/

/

Notes

top priorities for this week

_____

_____

_____

_____

_____

Victories for the week

looking ahead to next week

_____

_____

_____

_____

_____

_____

_____

_____

This Week

/

/

/

/

/

/

/

Notes

top priorities for this week

_____
_____
_____
_____
_____

Victories for the week

looking ahead to next week

_____
_____
_____
_____
_____
_____
_____
_____
_____

This Week

/

/

/

/

/

/

/

Notes

top priorities for this week

_____
_____
_____
_____
_____

Victories for the week

looking ahead to next week

_____
_____
_____
_____
_____
_____
_____
_____

This Week

_____

/

/

/

/

/

/

/

Notes

top priorities for this week

_____
_____
_____
_____
_____

Victories for the week

looking ahead to next week

_____
_____
_____
_____
_____
_____
_____

This Week

_____

_____

_____

_____

_____

_____

_____

_____

_____

_____

_____

_____

_____

_____

_____

_____

_____

_____

/

/

/

/

/

/

/

Notes

top priorities for this week

Victories for the week

looking ahead to next week

This Week

/

/

/

/

/

/

/

Notes

Victories for the week

looking ahead to next week

This Week

/

/

/

/

/

/

/

Notes

top priorities for this week

_____
_____
_____
_____
_____

Victories for the week

looking ahead to next week

_____
_____
_____
_____
_____
_____
_____
_____

This Week

_____

/

/

/

/

/

/

/

Notes

Victories for the week

looking ahead to next week

This Week

/

/

/

/

/

/

/

Notes

Victories for the week

looking ahead to next week

This Week

_____

_____

_____

_____

_____

_____

_____

_____

_____

_____

_____

_____

_____

_____

_____

_____

_____

_____

_____

_____

/

/

/

/

/

/

/

Notes

top priorities for this week

_____
_____
_____
_____
_____

Victories for the week

looking ahead to next week

_____
_____
_____
_____
_____
_____
_____

This Week

/

/

/

/

/

/

/

Notes

top priorities for this week

_____

_____

_____

_____

_____

_____

Victories for the week

looking ahead to next week

_____

_____

_____

_____

_____

_____

_____

_____

This Week

/

/

/

/

/

/

/

Notes

top priorities for this week

_____
_____
_____
_____
_____

Victories for the week

looking ahead to next week

_____
_____
_____
_____
_____
_____
_____

This Week

/

/

/

/

/

/

/

Notes

top priorities for this week

_____
_____
_____
_____
_____

Victories for the week

looking ahead to next week

_____
_____
_____
_____
_____
_____
_____

This Week

/

/

/

/

/

/

/

Notes

Victories for the week

looking ahead to next week

This Week

/

/

/

/

/

/

/

Notes

top priorities for this week

_____
_____
_____
_____
_____

Victories for the week

looking ahead to next week

_____
_____
_____
_____
_____
_____
_____
_____

This Week

/

/

/

/

/

/

/

Notes

top priorities for this week

Victories for the week

looking ahead to next week

This Week

_____
_____
_____
_____
_____
_____
_____
_____
_____
_____
_____
_____
_____
_____
_____
_____
_____
_____
_____
_____

/

/

/

/

/

/

/

Notes

Victories for the week

looking ahead to next week

This Week

/

/

/

/

/

/

/

Notes

top priorities for this week

_____

_____

_____

_____

_____

Victories for the week

looking ahead to next week

_____

_____

_____

_____

_____

_____

_____

_____

This Week

/

/

/

/

/

/

/

Notes

Victories for the week

looking ahead to next week

This Week

/

/

/

/

/

/

/

Notes

Victories for the week

looking ahead to next week

This Week

/

/

/

Notes

Victories for the week

looking ahead to next week

This Week

/

/

/

/

/

/

/

Notes

Victories for the week

looking ahead to next week

This Week

/

/

/

/

/

/

/

Notes

top priorities for this week

_____

_____

_____

_____

_____

Victories for the week

looking ahead to next week

_____

_____

_____

_____

_____

_____

_____

This Week

/

/

/

/

/

/

/

Notes

Victories for the week

looking ahead to next week

This Week

/

/

/

/

/

/

/

Notes

top priorities for this week

_____
_____
_____
_____
_____

Victories for the week

looking ahead to next week

_____
_____
_____
_____
_____
_____
_____

This Week

_____

/

/

/

/

/

/

/

Notes

top priorities for this week

Victories for the week

looking ahead to next week

This Week

/

/

/

/

/

/

/

Notes

top priorities for this week

_____
_____
_____
_____
_____

Victories for the week

looking ahead to next week

_____
_____
_____
_____
_____
_____
_____
_____

This Week

/

/

/

/

/

/

/

Notes

top priorities for this week

_____
_____
_____
_____
_____

Victories for the week

looking ahead to next week

_____
_____
_____
_____
_____
_____
_____

This Week

/

/

/

/

/

/

/

Notes

Victories for the week

looking ahead to next week

This Week

/

/

/

/

/

/

/

Notes

top priorities for this week

_____

_____

_____

_____

_____

Victories for the week

looking ahead to next week

_____

_____

_____

_____

_____

_____

_____

This Week

/

/

/

/

/

/

/

Notes

Victories for the week

looking ahead to next week

This Week

/

/

/

/

/

/

/

Notes

Victories for the week

looking ahead to next week

This Week

/

/

/

/

/

/

/

Notes

top priorities for this week

Victories for the week

looking ahead to next week

This Week

/

/

/

/

/

/

/

Notes

Victories for the week

looking ahead to next week

This Week

/

/

/

/

/

/

/

Notes

Victories for the week

looking ahead to next week

This Week

/

/

/

/

/

/

/

Notes

Victories for the week

looking ahead to next week

This Week

/

/

/

/

/

/

/

Notes

Victories for the week

looking ahead to next week

This Week

/

/

/

/

/

/

/

Notes

Victories for the week

looking ahead to next week

This Week

/

/

/

/

/

/

/

Notes

Victories for the week

looking ahead to next week

This Week

/

/

/

/

/

/

/

Notes

top priorities for this week

_____

_____

_____

_____

Victories for the week

looking ahead to next week

_____

_____

_____

_____

_____

_____

_____

This Week

/

/

/

/

/

/

/

Notes

Victories for the week

looking ahead to next week

This Week

/

/

/

/

/

/

/

Notes

top priorities for this week

_____
_____
_____
_____
_____

Victories for the week

looking ahead to next week

_____
_____
_____
_____
_____
_____
_____
_____

This Week

/

/

/

/

/

/

/

Notes

Victories for the week

looking ahead to next week

This Week

/

/

/

/

/

/

/

Notes

Victories for the week

looking ahead to next week

This Week

/

/

/

/

/

/

/

Notes

top priorities for this week

_____
_____
_____
_____
_____

Victories for the week

looking ahead to next week

_____
_____
_____
_____
_____
_____
_____

This Week

/

/

/

/

/

/

/

Notes

Victories for the week

looking ahead to next week

This Week

/

/

/

/

/

/

/

Notes

Victories for the week

looking ahead to next week

This Week

/

/

/

/

/

/

/

Notes

top priorities for this week

_____
_____
_____
_____
_____

Victories for the week

looking ahead to next week

_____
_____
_____
_____
_____
_____
_____

This Week

/

/

/

/

/

/

/

Notes

Victories for the week

looking ahead to next week

This Week

_____

/

/

/

/

/

/

/

Notes

top priorities for this week

_____

_____

_____

_____

_____

Victories for the week

looking ahead to next week

_____

_____

_____

_____

_____

_____

_____

_____

_____

This Week

/

/

/

/

/

/

/

Notes

Victories for the week

looking ahead to next week

This Week

/

/

/

/

/

/

/

Notes

Victories for the week

looking ahead to next week

This Week

/

/

/

/

/

/

/

Notes

top priorities for this week

_____
_____
_____
_____
_____

Victories for the week

looking ahead to next week

_____
_____
_____
_____
_____
_____
_____

Notes

Notes

Notes

Notes

Notes

Notes

Notes

Notes

Notes

Notes

Notes

Made in United States
Orlando, FL
14 April 2025

60539233R00070